DIET AND EXERCISE

expertise

Foreword

If you are a person who is looking for a way to make their life better and to make themselves feel better, diet and exercise are some good things to start with. Your diet and exercise routine has a large impact on the way your body will feel and function. It is important to consume only what you will burn off. A wide variety of food is suggested, you want to consume a little bit of everything in moderation. A couple things that are important to stay away from are saturated fat and trans fat.

It may be hard for you to stick to a diet and exercise routine, especially when it involves giving up some of your favorite foods. It is crucial that you do this if you wish to have a healthier body. It will take a great deal of commitment, dedication, and motivation, but it is possible. All you need is a source of information that you can use to guide you through the process of designing a diet and exercise routine. The following chapters in this book will provide you with information that will serve as your guide on your quest to a healthier mind, body, and spirit through dieting. Just make sure to pay close attention and retain all the information and you will surely realize how possible it is to begin a diet or begin exercising.

Diet and Exercise Expertise

Better Physical Personal Development Through Better Living

Table of Contents

Chapter 1:

Diet Basics

Synopsis

The idea of beginning a diet may seem like a daunting task. For most people it will be difficult to give up old easting habits and develop new ones. You need to keep in mind that not all diets are good diets.

You can actually cause more harm than good while adhering to certain diets. It is important that you have well balanced meals and you do not try to cut out necessary nutrients. Also, another important thing to remember is that people will often times make mistakes while on a diet. We are humans and none of us are perfect so therefore expect to have some slip ups every now and then.

If you are confused and do not know much about diets, do not worry, you are not alone. The following chapter will touch base on the basics of diets and provide you with helpful information that will put you off on a good start with your new diet.

The Basics

Eating a healthy diet is very important for the overall health and well-being of your body. Certain foods are packed with nutrients that are great for your body while others are packed with processed foods and sugars which are unhealthy for you.

For most people a serious diet will not be needed. The majority of people usually just need to cut a few things out of their current diet and replace them with a few new things. Some people may actually need intense diets with strict limits on carbs allowed per day as well as calories.

These types of foods should be limited with anybody, but those on strict diets can have almost none. There are many different diets and different diets work with different people. You just need to find the one that works for you and suits your needs.

The following are some examples of diets that can be dangerous and should be avoided:

Fad Diets:

It is important that you are aware of how dangerous fad diets can potentially be. In most cases these fad diets do more harm to the person than it does good. This is because fad diets usually involve nearly starving yourself. The amount of food a person is allowed to consume in these diets is usually quite minimal. Not only is it unhealthy to limit your food intake to ridiculous portions these fad diets also set many people up for failure.

This is because the person on the diet will likely continuously feel hungry. This will likely eventually lead to binge eating and eventually completely abandoning the diet. The problem with that is the fact that if you have been nearly starving yourself, your metabolism has greatly slowed down. Now you will notice that every little thing you eat packs more pounds on.

Many of these fad diets will also cause a person to feel weak and be more susceptible to certain illnesses. This is again due to the fact that most fad diets do not allow a person to consume all of the proper nutrients needed to produce energy throughout the day.

Tape Worms:

Can you believe that some people resort to eating tape worms to lose weight? Well you better start believing. This is actually starting to become quite a popular trend. This is probably due to the fact that people feel as if it is an easy way to diet. After all, they do not need to change their diet or limit their food consumption. Also, they will lose weight without exercising.

These seem like great benefits, right? Wrong! Consuming tape worms to lose weight is a terrible idea. It can be very damaging to a person's body. Tape worms are parasites which feed off of their host, which would be you.

Eating tape worms can lead to bloating, severe weight loss, nausea, vomiting, diarrhea, and loss of appetite. In severe cases can cause seizures, confusion, headaches, and even death! That does not sound like a beneficial diet to me, more like a death wish. Do not fall victim to the tape worm diet!

Cotton Ball Diet:

The name of this diet sounds crazy right? That is because it is crazy. It is exactly what it sounds like. Some people thought it would be a good idea to consume cotton balls in order to diet because they would make them feel full. Apparently their reasoning comes from the fact that cotton balls are low in calories. Well they are also extremely high in fiber which will likely lead to intestinal blockage over time. Sure they may lose weight, but it will be because they are in excruciating abdominal pain because their intestines are about to burst. This diet is a terrible idea and you should never try it!

Those were just a few examples of the countless dangerous diets that exist. Do not fall into trends and cause harm to your body. It is best to find a healthy balanced diet that works for you. The following chapters in this book will begin to go over how you should set your diet up in order to make it work for you and help you reach you goals of having a healthy body and a better life.

Chapter 2:

Synopsis

There are a few things that determine how many calories a person needs in order to maintain a healthy body. The number of calories that you should consume depends on your age, gender, height, and weight. The number of calories that a person needs to consume on a daily basis varies from person to person. Other factors need to be taken in to consideration while determining as well such as your level of daily activity. It is important that when you determine your number of allowed calories that you are sure that the calories you have consumed will be burned off during the day.

The following chapter will go further into detail about how many calories you should take in on a daily basis while dieting. Pay close information because the information provided will surely be helpful for you with your questions about calorie consumption.

Calorie Consumption While Dieting

There are several things to consider when designing a diet to limit calorie consumption. One of the most important is your level of activity. You do not want to deprive yourself of needed nutrients but at the same time you do not want to flood your body with calories that you cannot burn off. The best way to avoid this is do some basic math.

You must first figure out how many calories you currently burn per day. There are calculators on many health websites that are designed to help you with this process and make it much easier for you. Once you have determined how many calories you burn a day you begin the rest of the process of setting your calorie intake guidelines.

The next step is to figure out how many calories you need to consume regarding your current weight. If you are larger you need to consume fewer calories. Calories can easily turn into fat if not burned off during the day.so that is why it is important to limit them, especially if you are above average weight. At the same time, you cannot cut down your calorie intake too much because this will not have positive results.

If you are burning more than you are consuming your body will begin to burn muscle instead of fat. This is because fat cells serve as emergency reserves for your body so your body naturally tries to burn that last if it thinks it is malnourished.

After you have determined how many calories you need with your weight for your diet it is time to add in the age factor. Most adults need fewer calories than they did in their younger years. This is because most older adults are much less active than they were in their earlier years which leads to less calories being burned. As stated before, you do not want calories being left unburned in your body, they turn to fat. So if you are younger and active you will likely need to consume more calories but if you are older and less active less calories is the way to go.

Gender:

It is believed that men seem to need more calories on a day to day basis than women. This is due to the fact that men and women's bodies are different. We have different muscle structures from each other and therefore our bodies burn different amount of calories on a daily basis.

For example, an active male can require more than 3,000 calories a day when they are active. This means that they engage in sports or other activities which cause the body to work. The recommended intake for the average woman is 2,160 calories per day for an active woman. That is quite a big difference, isn't it?

Height:

This is pretty much common sense. If you are taller you are going to need more calories due to the fact that you have more body mass than shorter people. The more of you there is the more calories you need. Always remember, eating too many calories will lead to a gain in weight and setbacks in your diet. If you are trying to create a more healthy body and life for yourself then over indulging on calories is the last thing you want to do.

I hope that these tips on calorie consumption have been useful for you and have answered some of your questions. Keep in mind, diets need to be personalized to an individual's needs so what another person needs in calories will likely be different than you needs.

Trying to copy somebody else's diet because it works for them will likely have negative results for you since you will not be getting the balanced diet you need. There are also websites that have calorie calculators and these can help you greatly while you are trying to determine your number of needed daily calories.

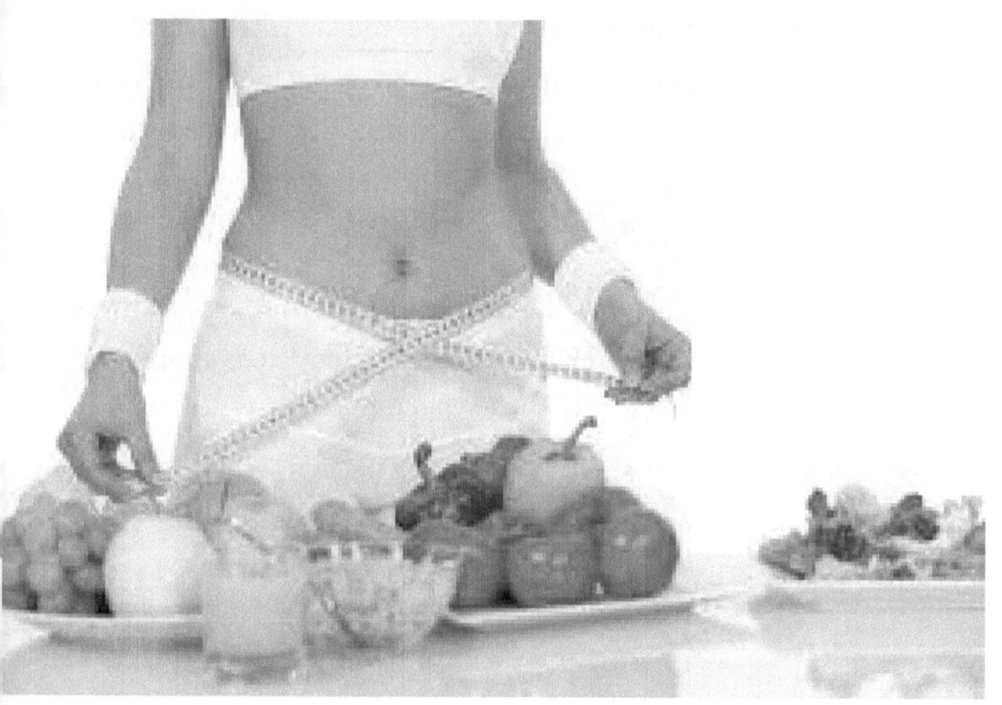

Chapter 3:

Synopsis

Are you tired of feeling sluggish or as if your body is just not up to par? Do you lack energy that you used to have? Do you find yourself tired and irritable more often than not? Do you have dark circles under your eyes? If you answered yes to any of these questions it is time for you to start eating a more healthy diet.

You need to have a diet consisting of well-balanced healthy foods and not a bunch of junk food garbage. The saying goes "you are what you eat" so therefore if you eat a bunch of crap food you are going to feel like crap. The same goes for healthy food. If you consume healthy foods on a regular basis as part of a healthy diet you will surely feel great and not have to deal with the side effects that unhealthy eating cause.

The following chapter will go a little further into detail about healthy eating and how it is related to a healthy body. Be sure to pay close attention and retain all information as it will surely be helpful for you.

Feel Better Through Dieting

If you are a person who has not felt quite like themselves for some time now and are not sure what is going on with your body, have you ever considered that it may be your diet? The food you consume determines the health of your body. If you constantly eat junk food your body will likely be in a low state of health. It will be easier for you to get sick and fight of illnesses, you will feel sick, low on energy, and sometimes even irritable. These are normal side effects of a poor diet. It only makes sense as our body needs certain nutrients to be able to function properly. If you rob your body of these essential nutrients it will do what it has to in order to make sure it makes it so see another day. In many cases, the body will cause undesirable side effects to itself in order to try to give you a hint that you need to start eating better.

Dieting can also be very beneficial for people facing certain mental strains in their current life. A proper diet can be very beneficial for the mental health of a person. Just like the rest of the human body, the brain needs certain essential nutrients in order to function properly. Not consuming a proper diet you will likely become easily stressed or overwhelmed as your brain will be deprived of the nutrients it needs to function.

It is your body and you only get one so you really need to take care of it. You need to remember that your body should be thought of as a temple and not a place that should be filled with bad things. Only let the best things in your body and keep the bad stuff away. I know this is easier said than done but with effort and determination it is possible.

Chapter 4:

Healthy Recipes

Synopsis

This chapter is meant to provide you with some valuable information on healthy recipes. We will go over a few examples of popular healthy recipes. This should give you an idea of what type of meals you will need to add to your diet to begin feeling healthier and to have a healthier mind, body, and spirit.

Keep in mind, eating healthy does not necessarily mean eating food that is tasteless or food that you do not like. There are many different types of meals that you can make that if prepared the right way can be very nutritious and healthy. You would likely be surprised by the countless number of options that are available. Many people think that going on a diet means that you have to give up all good food, this is not true! It simply means that you need to find more healthy alternatives for your current eating habits, you can find other things you like.

The following chapter contains recipes that you should not only find tasty but helpful for your diet as well.

Ideas for Healthy Recipes

It order for a meal to be considered healthy it generally needs to consist of 350 or less calories for the main portion of the dish. It should also contain 20 grams or less of fat and 5 grams or less of saturated fat. This is a general rule and can change from person to person depending on their body type and current health condition. Also, if your doctor sets a different diet for you it is important that you listen to what they say as they are trained professionals.

The following are some examples of some meals that follow the above guidelines:

Green Bean and Paprika Shrimp Sauté:

This is a delicious dish that bursts with flavor. It is sure to be a favorite for the whole family. The best part about this meal is that you will not even realize that you are eating diet friendly food. The dish is simple to prepare and the green beans add a snap and a bit of crunch to spruce the dish up. This is a Spanish inspired dish so it should be served with brown rice. You want this dish to be somewhat garlicky for best results, It may also be served with quinoa. You may want to consider purchasing pre-peeled shrimp. They may be more expensive but they do come with the convenience of saving a lot of time.

Chopped Salad al Tonno:

If you are looking for something light that won't drag you down for the rest of the day, chopped salad al tonno is perfect for you. This salad is much better than a boring tuna sandwich and also gets rid of the problem of carbs from bread. It is not difficult to make and does not take many ingredients. The total prep time is about 15 minutes so it is quick to prepare as well. All you need to do is stir together some lemon, salt and pepper, garlic, and oil in a large bowl. Once everything is mixed together add olives, romaine lettuce, tomatoes and olives and then toss to coat. Once you have done this you add tuna and toss again. This salad makes an awesome lunch but can be good for a snack as well.

Grilled Egg Plant Panini:

This is another great treat this is very healthy and can be enjoyed by the whole family. Presentation is important with this dish because you do not want it to look sloppy. Once again this is not a complicated dish to complete and only takes about 35 minutes.

It is important while shopping for your egg plants to look for ones that do not have mushy spots. They also need to be nice and purple and be medium in size. The best time to find egg plants like this is toward the end of summer. To prepare this dish you simply combine a small amount of mayonnaise and basil in a bowl.

Then you lightly brush each side of the eggplant of one tablespoon of oil as well as one side of each piece of bread. You then need to grill the eggplant on medium high for approximately 6 minutes. Flip the eggplant and top with cheese. Grill for approximately four more minutes or until cheese is melted and the eggplant is tender. After that you need to grill toast the bread by grilling it about one to two minutes. All that is left now is to put your sandwiches together! Simply place the eggplant on the toasted bread, cheesy side up, and top with red peppers, some onion, and the other piece of bread. Enjoy!

Baby Tiramisu:

If you are like most people, even though you are dieting you still want the occasional treat of some sweets. A baby tiramisu is a perfect solution for this problem. To create this splendid dish you will need to combine a half cup of non-fat ricotta cheese and two tablespoons of confectioners' sugar in a bowl. You will then need to add a half of a teaspoon of vanilla extract. Also mix in an eight teaspoon of ground cinnamon.

All you need to do then is place your lady fingers in an appropriate sized baking dish and drizzle two tablespoons of expresso over them. Then you spread your ricotta mixture over the lady fingers. After you have done this you need to place another lady finger on top of the ricotta mixture and pour another two tablespoons of expresso evenly over them. You then need to drizzle with two tablespoons of melted chocolate, bittersweet chocolate chips are recommended.

Chapter 5:

Exercise Basics

Synopsis

A healthy diet is not the only thing that is important in having a healthier body and mind. It is also important to make sure that you are also getting the right amount of exercise.

At first it may be difficult to get yourself in the routine of exercising on a regular basis. With practice and determination you will find yourself doing it in no time. You will be amazed by how much better you feel every day when you exercise on a regular basis.

Exercise will not only provide you with a healthy body and mind; it will also increase the span of your life. This will give you many extra years to spend with your loved ones.

The following chapter will touch base on the basics of exercise and why exercise is so important while dieting.

The Basics on Exercise

Many people make the error of thinking that a proper diet alone is enough to achieve full body health. This is not the case! A well balanced diet also needs to include regular exercise as this is vital for a person to be healthy.

Exercising will also give you the added benefit of being able to eat more food on a daily basis. While you exercise you burn off fat and calories. The more calories you burn the more you will be able to eat. As well, it will be more acceptable for you to step outside of your diet plan on occasion when you are exercising. After all, you deserve the occasional treat.

Exercise will not only get your body to a better physical state, it will also make you feel better mentally as well. Did you know that your brain naturally releases endorphins while you exercise? When your brain is full of endorphins you will achieve a state of euphoria or a type of high that will make you feel good.

You will feel great about yourself as you begin to see the results from all the effort you have out into your exercise routine. It will make you a more confident person and it will improve your self-worth and self-respect. This will lead to many new great doors opening in your life and ample opportunities. The first thing you need in order to have a happy successful life is a healthy body, spirit, and mind. Exercise can greatly help to improve the state of each one of these.

There is always time to exercise so do not give yourself any excuses. You do not need to do a hour long routine. Doing what you can with the time you have will help. Any effort is still effort.

Chapter 6:

Synopsis

Once you have decided to begin exercising it is important to set up a exercise routine for yourself. This will allow you to make sure that you are getting proper amounts of exercise while exercising different muscle groups and giving you a schedule to stick to.

You need to remember that nobody is going to hold you accountable for bot sticking to that routine but yourself. Slacking off or procrastinating when it comes to your exercise routine will do nothing but slow down the progress of your results which will likely suck your motivation to continue dry.

The following chapter will give you some helpful hints about how to set up a beneficial exercise routine and some important points to consider while doing so.

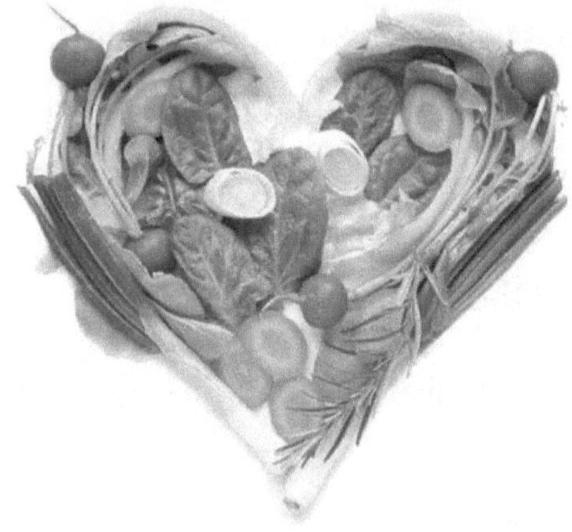

Create a Beneficial Routine

It is important that you do not try to start your journey to a healthier body and exercise blindly. You need to know some important facts so that you do not injure yourself while trying to better yourself. After all, you do not want to take one step forward and two steps back, do you? I didn't think so. It is always a good idea to consult a trained professional when developing an effective workout routine. These professionals will know the exact routine that will work best with the time you have available, your body type, and the goals that you have in mind.

For those who decide not to use a professional to build their exercise routine, you need to make sure you create a well-balanced exercise routine. You do not want to focus on one muscle group and work on it every day. This can damage muscles over time as they do not have enough time to heal properly. You need to work on different muscle groups on different days of the week. For example, one day you may work on biceps and then the next you work on legs.

If you are exercising for dieting purposes you may want to stick to exercises that focus more on the cardio aspect of things. Treadmills and step climbers can be great ways of burning off carbs and calories. The only problem is the fact that they take up so much space. Most people will not have room in their house for a treadmill so they may have to buy a gym membership. Stationary cycles are also another form of healthy cardio exercises. This type of cardio can be great for older people or those with arthritis as it allows the person working out to sit and take things at their own pace.

There are classes that even incorporate dancing into the cycling to provide an intense workout that is also fun.

If you find yourself having a hard time with sticking to your exercise routine you may want to try adding in some classes that you find fun. The dance exercise craze is exploding and you can find classes for this type of exercise almost anywhere. Programs like Zumba Dance can be quite fun so they hold you attention and bring you back for more and more. During these classes you will have so much fun that you do not even realize you are sweating and burning fat and calories.

Some older individuals may have a hard time bearing weight on their joints. There are special exercise routines that these people can utilize. One example of a form of exercise these older people can still participate in is water aerobics. These water aerobics usually take place in a swimming pool and allow people to exercise without bearing too much weight on their joints. You would be surprised by how well this form of exercise actually works. There is also the option of using workout equipment with counter weights on it. This option is used many times for physical rehabilitation from injuries. It allows the muscles to be strained enough to get exercise but not enough force to damage the persons joints or muscles.

No matter what your exercise goals are, they are accomplishable. All you need to do is find something that you enjoy doing as exercise and before you know it, you will begin to see positive results.

Chapter 7:

Synopsis

The biggest problem that you will face on your journey to a healthier body through diet and exercise will likely be to stay motivated. It can be difficult to continue with your journey at times but it is essential for a better life. Staying motivated is vital if you want to stick to your plans.

The following chapter will provide you with some helpful idea on how to stay motivated and to continue with your diet and exercise routine.

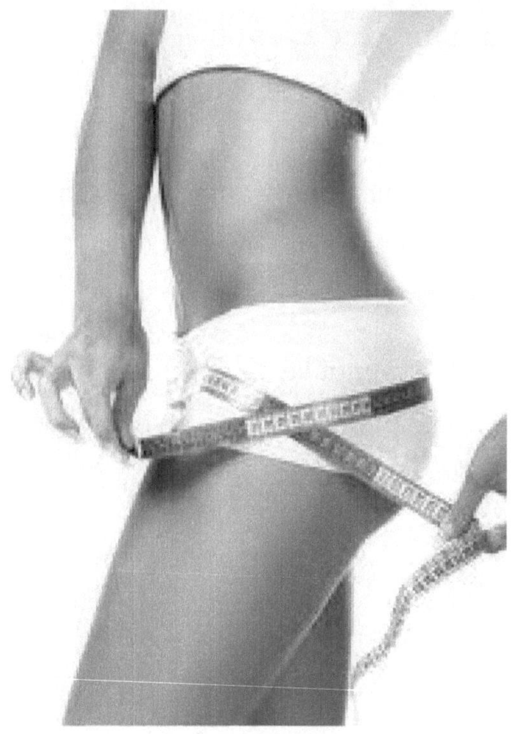

Keep it Going!

One thing that will surely help to keep you motivated is to think of all the hard effort and time you have spent on getting as far as you have with your diet and exercise routine. You do not want to throw it all away do you? Of course not! You need to give yourself credit for the accomplishments you have made so far as well as your progress towards your future goals.

Another good idea is to use your family and friends as a way to keep you motivated. It can be difficult to hold yourself accountable at time because your mind naturally likes to minimize things. Your family and friends can be a good source of honest feedback. Your loved ones and friends will also have a large impact on your thinking if they think that you are starting to lose your motivation. In some cases other people can actually motivate you more than yourself. This is especially true if your health is at risk if you do not continue your diet. Your loved ones should remind you of how much they love you and how much they want you to be healthy. This will make you feel selfish if you start to slack on your diet or exercise and this will likely make you want to get back on track.

Some things in this life cannot be accomplished by you on your own and it is ok to reach out for help. Remember, you do not want to go back to square one so catch yourself quickly if you slip so you do not have to climb all the way back up again.

Wrapping Up

Bettering your life through a healthy diet and proper exercise is possible. Remember, you can do anything that you set your mind to. You deserve to have a healthy body, spirit, and mind. The only one who can provide it to you is you. Start working on a brighter future for yourself today and begin eating healthier foods and exercising regularly. You will not be disappointed with the results. Keep in mind, great effort is rewarded with great results.

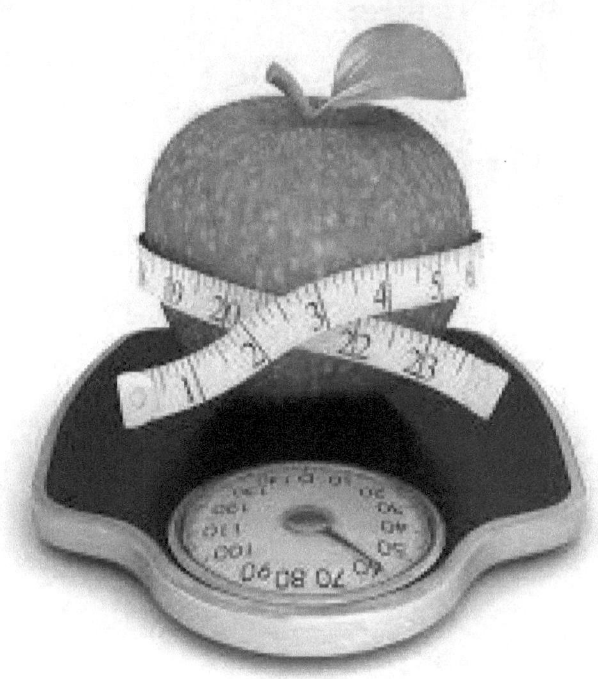

Eating Healthy

All The Info On Eating For A Healthy Life

Table Of Contents

Foreword

In simple terms the body has two very different and complex systems of energy producing sources. As energy is vital to the very existence of human activity and survival the two energy style depend on each other for support. This book shows you what foods give you the most energy.

It occurs so very frequently - we resolve to go on with a health and physical fitness program with zest and likely much fanfare too; however in the first week of going into the plan, everything peters out.

Why is it that we don't stick with the diet plans, the morning jogging plans, the physical exercise plans that we make?

And what may we do to ensure we keep going with these plans, for our own sake and for the sake of the individuals that are dependent on us?

Are you eating simply to satisfy your appetite or to make your taste buds happy? Or are you eating in order to take better command of your life? In this eBook, we see how you are able to make your life much more optimal simply by making a point that you eat correctly.

Eating Healthy
All The Info On Eating For A Healthy Life

Chapter 1:

The Basics

Synopsis

Energy is needed for the various functions like maintenance of growth, daily activities, exercise and many other movements or functions that are often taken for granted. These are shared between the two energy systems.

In today's world, seldom do any health and fitness plans work. What's the reason for their alarming rate of failure?

The world is a lot less healthful than it was two decades ago. Much this is attributed to the altered food habits of individuals.

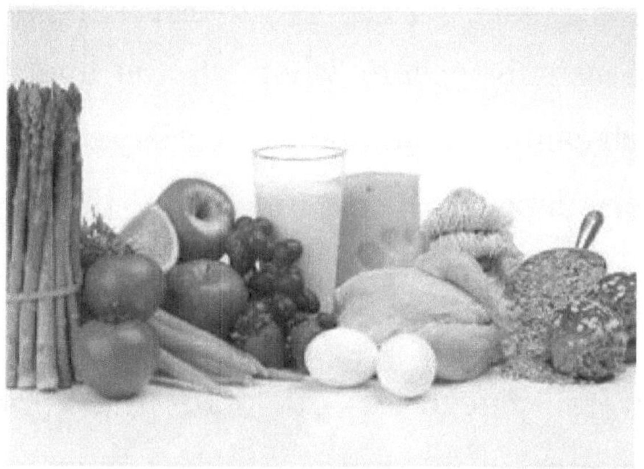

The Basics

The primary and first to be used energy system is the aerobic system. This system uses oxygen for the function of the muscles and does demand quite a lot from the general body system.

This demand usually increases the rate and depth of breathing and blood supply mainly because of the corresponding increase of the heart rate.

When the body requires more energy which cannot be met due to the elevated need for more oxygen then the body system automatically switched to the anaerobic energy system. This system is able to produce energy without the need to use oxygen.

All this energy is generated through the suitable or correct consumption of foods. The foods consumed dictate the types of energy levels each individual is capable of producing.

Muscle fatigue usually occurs when all the energy sources are exhausted which can be attributed to a variety of reasons; the most compelling one depends very much on the types of foods consumed.

There are several categories of foods that produce various beneficial elements for the human body system and noting the ones that create or enhance the energy generating sources is definitely useful to know. Therefore this knowledge should help the individual choose the right types of foods.

The aerobic system works by breaking down the carbohydrates, fatty acids and amino acids in the foods consumed while the anaerobic system releases energy from the foods stored in the body, usually during intense activity bouts.

If we hear about the failure of diets or gym plans all around us, commonly it isn't their fault. Commonly it is the fault of the individuals who started with much commotion about going through these plans, telling all their acquaintances and co-workers about it, and then didn't abide by those programs.

The individuals who abandon the exercise or diet halfway do not see the advantages, naturally, and everybody blames the plan.

What the world needs nowadays isn't a fresh health or fitness program or a diet, but it requires motivation. It needs the correct sort of mind-set to follow through with whatever plan they have chosen to the very end.

If they can do that, most of the health issues that are related to life-style situations will get to be outmoded. And we don't have to visit the corners of the earth to discover this motivation. The motivation lies right here, inside us; we simply need to search it out and utilize it.

One generation ago, individuals wouldn't dream of picking up whatever junk food they could get in order to feed their faces. Nowadays, we do that so very casually. "I'm hungry" commonly means "I want a burger or a hot dog, likely with chips on the side and some cola." And, "I am on a diet" means "I am on a chemically ridden pill which will defeat my hunger and deprive my body of vitamins." It's genuinely no wonder that we are facing so many health issues today.

Our health is an indicator of what we consume. The sorry condition that we're living in isn't an individual problem; it's a global issue. The world as a whole is eating incorrectly. Six in every ten individuals in the US is overweight, and the number is going to be eight in every ten individuals by the time we hit 2015.

Are we truly thinking about this? We aren't. Even as you're studying this eBook, you likely have a packet of chips on the side. Do you know that what you spent on that package, which is filling your stomach with some of the most toxic chemicals known to humanity, could instead have fed an emaciated youngster in Ruanda?

But it's not simply about being philanthropic. It's about ourselves too. Yes, we have to be selfish. With such appalling health figures, aren't we heading for doom? We're definitely not eating right. Whatever excess baggage that brings - obesity and the assorted ill health in its wake - we have to be prepared for it.

So the next time you see that a program has failed or is receiving a lot of criticism, remember that the criticism isn't probably because the program stands on shaky ground. In most cases, it is because people began with great intentions and then did not follow the program as they should have

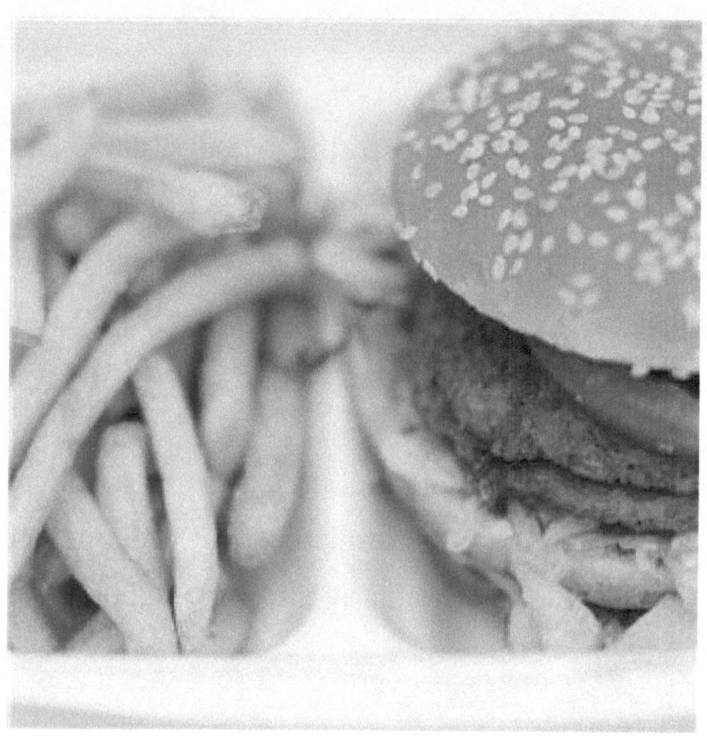

Chapter 2:

Synopsis

The most crucial thing that you need to keep your health and fitness program alive - even more crucial than an instructor or a doctor - is your own motive.

You have to be determined to scrutinize the situation. So, you're overweight and are looking at casting off a few pounds. No gym instructor from anyplace in the world will help you if you don't take adequate measures to have the right diet and to stick to your routine exercise.

Even if you're sick and are looking at treatment, no physician will help if you aren't determined in following the treatment platform, whether it's taking the medication at the correct time or abstaining from some foods.

Your Mindset

We have strayed horribly with our eating habits thus far. Unless we take stock of the state of affairs and take matters in our own hands, matters are not going to get better.

The number 1 thing is awareness. We have to learn what foods are correct for us and what are not. We have to go back to training and comprehend what the nutrients are that your body truly wants and in what amount.

Then we have to build a dietary regimen for ourselves and our loved ones so that we eat healthier. We have to cut down on all the foods that are adverse - the sugars, the fats, the carbohydrates, we don't truly want them - and incorporate foods that may boost our health.

This does sound too preachy, I understand. But that's the only reprieve we have got. If we continue munching on Oreos, we're never going to get better.

But there's hope. Hope lies in the fact that there are a lot of foods out there that are simply as tasty as those awful junk foods but we don't yet know about them.

These are the foods that we don't know about yet, we likely don't care for them or as we don't know how to fix them, but a healthy cookbook may help you in understanding assorted interesting ways to healthy cooking.

Even with the same sort of diet you eat, you are able to conjure up some really delicious healthy dishes. Yes, it's all very much possible. You are able to modify your eating habits to a big extent, while at the same time attending to your palate.

The fact is that the weight loss industry is responsible in a really significant way towards this downfall of the developed human race. They have to keep selling their Atkinses and Jenny Craigs and Zones and Medifasts and for that reason the media never tells you how we may in reality take things in your own hands.

They show us glitzy before-after pictures of a person with a foot-long sub and then the same guy with 6 pack abs and tell us that the diet made that possible.

However the fact is, if we were to get our head together, we may very easily do that too, without having to spend 1000s of dollars on those diets. And what do we have to do?

2 general things:-

Control what we consume.
Indulge in physical exertion.

Now, is that too much to accomplish? Don't we owe that to our body that has served us so well all these years? Don't we owe that to ourselves and our loved ones?

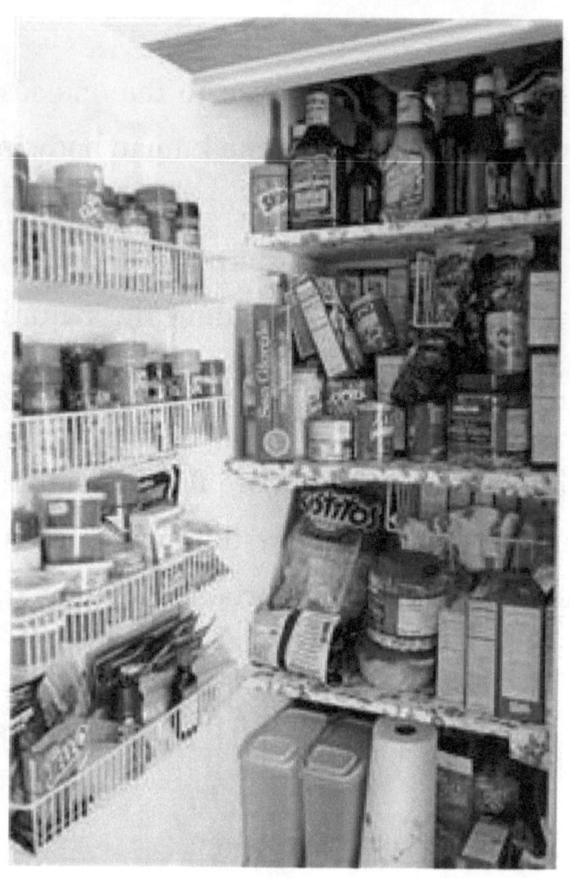

Chapter 3:
Honey And Whole Grains

Synopsis

Over the years honey has been proven to the one sustaining power behind the energy circle. Benefiting the human body in various areas it is foremost still unrivaled in its energy producing entity. Honey is nature's most natural energy booster. It also acts as an effective immunity system builder while providing the natural remedy to a host of varied ailments too.

Energy is very important to the smooth flowing natural of a daily life cycle of any human being. Therefore finding energy sources that are both consistent and healthy are important to keeping fit and happy.

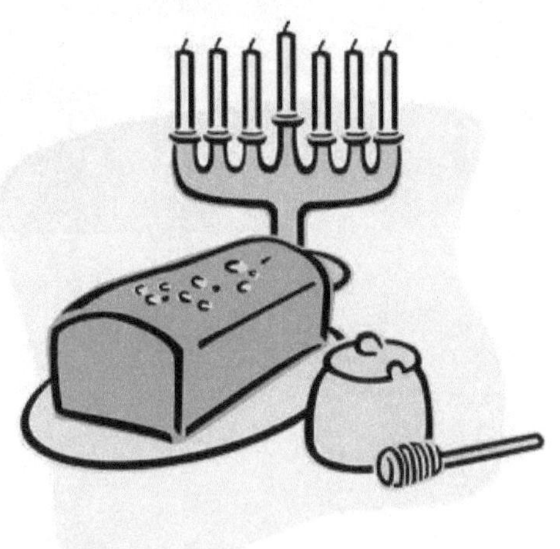

A Good Pair

The natural benefits of honey has been widely acknowledged and accepted. Besides its great taste, honey is also a natural source of carbohydrate, which is an energy maker for boosting performance, endurance and reducing levels of muscle fatigue.

This is especially useful for athletes. The sugar content in the honey helps to play a role in preventing fatigue during exercise sessions and also during training sessions for sports enthusiast. These sugar make ups are divided into glucose and fructose and functions in different but complimenting ways.

The glucose content in the honey is generally absorbed at a faster rate and gives off an immediate energy boost while the fructose works at a slower pace for a more sustainable and prolonged energy dispersement. When it comes to addressing blood sugar levels in the body system, honey has been known to help keep the levels fairly constant.

As honey is a pleasant food product and it's natural in its form, consuming it is not a very difficult exercise. People of all ages are generally quite willing to consume honey in any of its accompanying forms. It's even popular with children.

The energy produced from consuming a small amount of honey daily helps children cope with the physical strains of daily school activities and sports commitments. For the adults too consuming a daily small dose of honey can go a long way in keeping the energy levels at its best during a demanding day at work.

Making sandwiches with honey accompanied with other fillings is one way of creating a pleasant snack. Applying honey on a freshly toasted slice of bread is also a welcome breakfast alternative. Adding honey to drinks instead of using sugar is definitely encouraged.

Most people today want a quick fix for their energy boosting needs and this usually comes in the unhealthy forms of sports drinks, coffee and refined carbohydrates like sugar and while bread.

Though these produce the desired heightened energy levels, it should be noted that this energy is fairly short lived and the tiredness that follows is usually more acutely felt. Therefore opting to consume some form of whole grains is not only a better alternative but is also much healthier.

Whole grains provide the energy that comes in a more complex form which breaks down over a longer period of time. This then creates the platform for sustaining the energy levels for longer periods.

Because of its more complex make up the whole grains come with a array of beneficial elements like minerals, vitamins, phytonutrients and fiber which are also rich in fiber.

Adding the whole grain ingredients is any dish more often than not completes the flavor or enhances it altogether. Whole grains can the various forms such as wheat, oat, barley, maize, brown rice, faro, spelt, emmer, einkorn, rye, millet, buckwheat, and many more.

These can then be made into various other products like whole wheat flour, whole wheat bread, whole wheat pasta, rolled oats or oat groats, triticale flour, popcorn and teff flour.

The benefits of consuming whole grains consistently can help decrease the risk of heart disease, lower cholesterol levels protect against many types of cancer and assist in weight management. Whole grains should not be confused with its lesser and more refined "cousin". Though refined grains have some benefits it is always better to opt for the whole grain alternatives

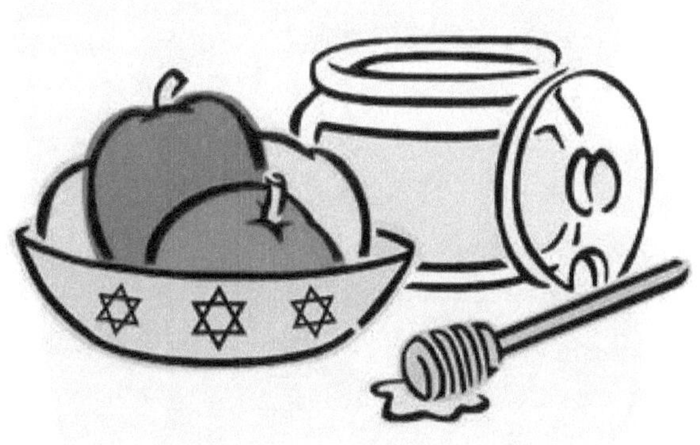

Chapter 4:

Nuts And Lean Meat

Synopsis

Nuts are an important source of nutrients for both human and animal consumption. Being rich in a whole host of necessary nutrients it can be eaten in its raw form, cooked or as an additive to already pre existing dishes. Thought nuts are defined as a hard shelled fruit, there are many other foods that are included in the nut family.

Different types of meats generally contribute to a variety of flavors; however the healthiest type is the one with as much lean meat content as possible. Its undisputed fact that the meats that contain a good amount of fat are a culinary treat indeed but for health purposes taking the time to understand the benefits of consuming lean meats is very wise indeed.

Good Proteins And Oils

It is now common knowledge that nuts greatly help in keeping a lot of ailments in check or from occurring at all. For instance, nuts have been known to be able to keep the possibility of coronary heart diseases manifesting, even for those whole come from a long line of family members with this problem.

Consuming nuts like almonds and walnuts have been known to lower serum cholesterol concentrations within the body system. Nuts are also highly recommended for those individuals suffering from insulin resistance problems like diabetics.

Turning to nuts rather that junk food to quell cravings is also another healthier alternative. Containing essential fatty acids is also another plus point when it comes to choosing nuts as a healthier alternative. Because nuts are healthy and can be consumed in its raw form, it is also another added advantage to keeping these around and handy as snacks.

Almonds are often used to normalize blood lipids because of their slow burn characteristics, which help to keep the blood sugar levels consistently healthy. Rich in a varied amount of different nutrients the almond is a popular additive to the stale diet of most Mediterranean people.

The Brazil nut is also another nutritious nut which comes with its own set of benefits when consumed in moderation. Noted for its omega 3 fatty acid content, the Brazil nut is also a good source of calcium.

Cashew nut is another very popular nut that is often consumed as a salted snack. However it would be a much healthier food product without the addition of salt, as it is already quite a flavorful nut on its own. In some parts of the world these nuts are made into oils.

The selection process should be done with a little knowledge as depending solely on what the naked eye perceives is not enough. Generally lean meats derived from beef cuts should include round, chuck, sirloin and tenderloin, while the cuts from pork or lamb would constitute tenderloin, loin chops and leg. The leanest parts of the poultry would be the breast area without the skin.

Though there are many reasons people eliminate meat from their daily diet, there is no evidence to show that this is a good or bad choice not should it be followed by all.

However the important point to note here is the choice of the types of meats that would make the consumption healthy and this would generally mean meats with lesser amount of fat content. Though white meat is by no means lacking in fat content, it is by comparison much less in fat content than red meats.

The nutritional value of consuming lean meats is quite extensive and rounded. Lean meats have a generally higher and purer content of protein which is a very important contributing factor to fundamental structural and functional progress of every cell sustenance and formation.

Lean meats are also a good source of essential amino acids particularly sulphur amino acids. When compared to the digestive rates the proteins in meats work faster than the one contained in the beans and whole wheat range.

Lean meat is also a good source of iron. Because iron deficiency is progressive it is often not detected until a later stage where anemia has developed.

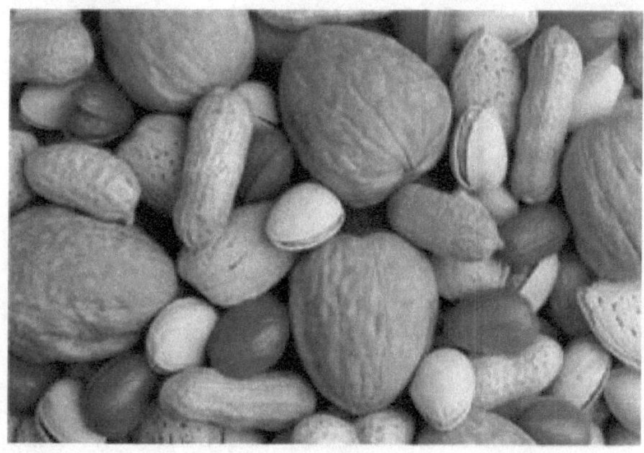

Chapter 5:

The Benefits

Synopsis

Here is all the motive you'd require to continue eating healthy.

Let's immediately plunge into the subject.

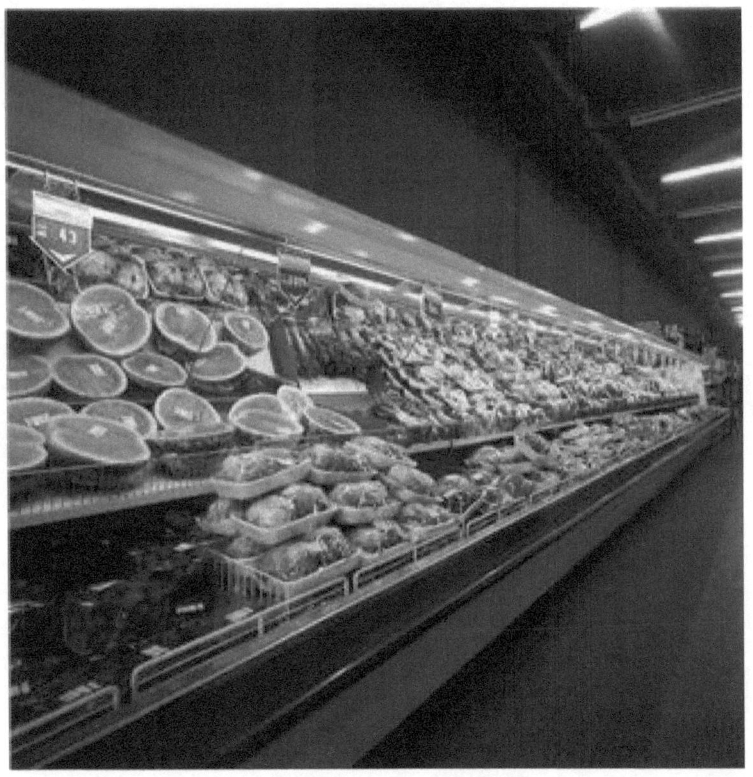

Advantages

You Get Healthier

We might whole collection of books about the health advantages of eating correctly and still it wouldn't quite cover what advantages genuinely exist. The most important advantage is that you gain command over your weight.

By eating correctly, you likewise make certain that your metabolic functions - most notably your immune system and your gastrointestinal system - keep working correctly. You're likewise protected from assorted chronic diseases, right from cardiovascular diseases like coronary artery disease and high blood pressure to diabetes.

More Cost Effective

Eating healthy means you spend much less. Your bills at the supermarkets come down drastically and you don't plunge farther into charge card debt if that is already an issue with you. In addition to that, you save a huge bundle on all the healthcare expenses you'd need if any issue surfaces because of your food binging habits.

Less Toxins In Your Body

A lot of foods nowadays are toxic because of the synthetic chemicals present in them. When you're attempting to eat correctly, you are much less likely to get these toxins into your body as one of the basic dogmas of eating correctly is that you shouldn't eat anything that's man-made.

In addition to that, if you eat less, you'll likewise be able to reduce on vices like smoking and alcoholism. A glass of beer is almost synonymous with a night out with the boys. If you eat less, you won't want the beer as well. Similarly, you will not want that one (or more) mandatory smoke that you tend to have after each meal.

More Physical Lifestyle

When you eat better, you'll find that you are able to do your work in a much better way. You are able to exercise more, travel more, play more, work more and therefore make your life more productive.

That sure beats being a fat slob and lounging around on the couch the whole day, doesn't it? You are able to also be more involved with your friends and loved ones and that surely enriches your life.

Good Social Life

Forget about fat fetishism, individuals who are overweight don't look appealing. There's a strong social taboo about weight on the wrong places of the body. If you're trying to find a partner, your flab may literally get in the way. Not simply that, individuals who can't control their eating habits and hence their weight are looked down upon by society as being individuals who can't control their basic urges.

This sort of psychology does exist, though very few individuals will speak about it. When you eat correctly, you'll discover that such issues disappear.

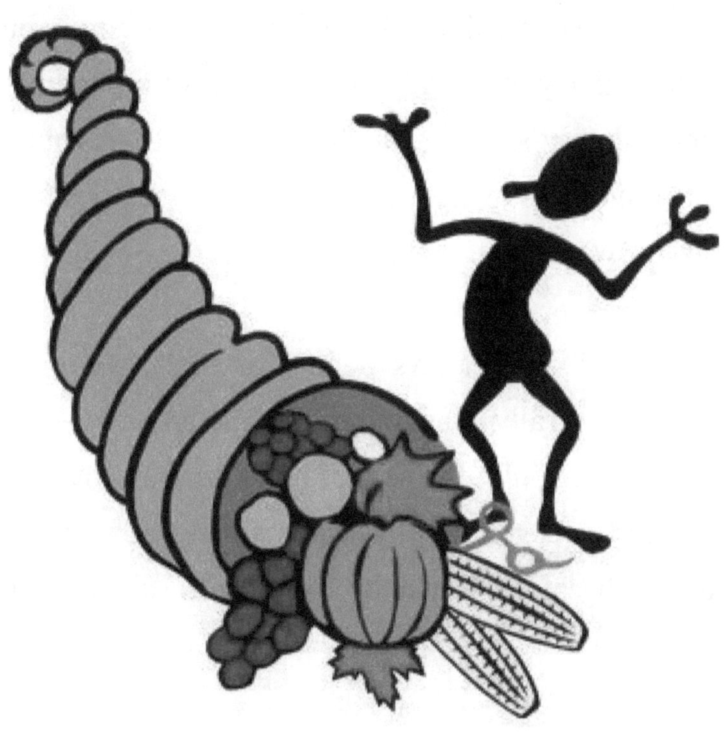

Wrapping Up

There are a lot of popular diets on the market nowadays, but most of them are unhealthy and occasionally even unsafe. This will explain how to eat a healthy, balanced diet for life and keep away from unhealthy diets.

Ascertain how many calories your body requires to function every day.

This number may vary wildly, depending on your metabolism and how physically active you are. If you're the sort of individual who puts on ten pounds simply smelling a slice of pizza, then your every day caloric intake ought to stay approximately 2000 calories for men, and 1500 calories for women.

Your body mass likewise plays a part in that: More calories are appropriate for naturally bigger individuals, and fewer calories for littler individuals. If you're the sort of individual who can eat without gaining a pound, or you're physically active, you might wish to increase your daily caloric intake by 1000-2000 calories, a bit less for women.

Don't dread fatty foods.

You have to consume fat from foods for your body to run correctly. But, it's crucial to pick out the correct sorts of fats: Most animal fats and a few vegetable oils are high in the sort of fats that raise your LDL cholesterol levels; the foul cholesterol.

Different than popular belief, eating cholesterol doesn't inevitably bring up the amount of cholesterol in your body. If you provide your body the correct tools, it will flush extra cholesterol from your body. Those tools are monounsaturated fatty acids, which you ought to try to consume regularly. Foods that are rich in monounsaturated fatty acids are olive oil, nuts, fish oil, and assorted seed oils.

Eat plenty of the correct carbs.

You have to eat foods high in carbs since they're your body's chief source of energy. The trick is to pick out the correct carbs. Simple carbs like sugar and refined flour are quickly absorbed by the body's gastrointestinal system.

This induces a sort of carb overload, and your body releases vast amounts of insulin to battle the overload. Not only is the excess insulin bad on your heart, however it encourages weight gain. Eat plenty of carbs, but consume carbs that are slowly digested by the body such as whole grain flour, veggies, oats, and unprocessed grains.

Eat bigger meals early on in the day.

Your metabolism decelerates toward the end of the evening and is less efficient at digesting foods. That means more of the power stored in the food will be stacked away as fat and your body won't absorb as many nutrients from the meal. Try eating a medium-sized meal for breakfast, a big meal for lunch, and a little meal for dinner. Better yet, attempt consuming 4-6 small meals over the run of your day.

Provide yourself a cheat meal.

Cheating doesn't mean gorging on all the wrong foods once a week; it implies enjoying a food you truly love once a week. Have a couple slices of pizza on Sundays, or a huge slice of double chocolate cake on Saturdays. This cheat meal will help you stick with the change in diet, and in a few ways it's really good for your body. Special occasions, like birthdays in the family, count as cheat meals.

Get the habit of eating slowly.

It will satisfy you with fewer calories and will forestall overeating and obesity with all its consequences.

Drink plenty of H2O.

It makes you feel more awake and energized, does wonders for your skin and makes you feel fuller so you wind up eating less! Cutting down soda and replacing it with water will do wonders for you.